Table of Contents

How To Portion Control For Weight Loss (Without Starving!)

Are you struggling to lose weight or looking for an easier way to eat healthy without feeling hungry all the time? Portion control is a great method to lose weight and monitor your healthy eating. This post explains what portion control is and offers tons of tips for how to successfully portion control yourself to healthy!

Portion control is one of the biggest nutrition hacks I've found for sticking to a healthy lifestyle, losing weight, and then maintaining my ideal weight. The idea is to understand what your body needs and just eat to that level. Oftentimes, either because we feel we have to finish all that's on our plate or restaurants have pre-determined giant portions, we over-eat, which leads to weight gain.

Enter portion control, which helps us to identify what's in our food and how much we need to consume to meet our goals. The hang-up for many people when trying lo lose weight, however, is they think they need to drastically reduce the amount of food they're eating, which isn't necessarily the case. My goal in this post is to share how to portion control without feeling hungry all the time, and still lose the weight (assuming that's your goal). The bottom line is that portion control means no food is off limits — it's just a matter of choice if and when you choose to eat anything.

Hopefully, the info I have shared below will help provide you some much needed support and control over this process. In a nutshell, here are the portion control topics we're gonna cover in this post:

WHY IS PORTION CONTROL IMPORTANT?

In basic terms, your body requires a certain amount of calories to function and survive each day. Those calories are determined by your age, current weight, and daily activity level and vary from person to person. An average woman requires approximately 2000 calories per day to maintain her weight, and 1500 calories per day to lose one pound of weight per week. An average man, on the other hand, requires approximately 2500 calories per day to maintain his weight, and 2000 to lose one pound of weight per week.

That's where portion control comes in. If you're eating more calories than your body needs, your body will take those extra calories and store them as fat. The more extra calories you consumer, the more fat you'll store.

So, in order to reduce those extra calories being stored as fat, we can use portion control to make sure we are eating what our body actually needs.

The reason why this is so difficult for many of us to do is we are constantly provided with larger portions than we need. This causes us to eat more without even realizing we've over-eaten, causing weight gain.

HOW PORTION CONTROL CAN HELP YOU LOSE WEIGHT

By portioning out our food and controlling the amounts of food we put into our bodies, we can essentially assume control over how much of our food will be stored as fat. And, if we eat at a calorie deficit, which means we eat less than what our body requires each day to function, we can then make our body use stored fat for energy, which causes weight loss. The more stored fat your body burns, the more weight you lose, up to a point, which is why we want to make sure we maintain a healthy, balanced diet while we utilize portion control.

10 PORTION CONTROL TIPS FOR HOW TO GET STARTED

Don't worry, this isn't where I suggest you eat carrot sticks and celery al day to lose weight. In fact, I recommend eating portions that make you feel full and satisfied, all the while understanding the food breakdown of what you're eating. To help you, I've gathered some portion control tips that helped me when I first started.

1. Read all nutrition labels. This is a biggie and will definitely be a big help to understand what's in your food. It's so important to read the labels to understand serving sizes. This doesn't mean we then go by what the label recommends as a serving, however. Instead, we use labels to understand how much of that food we should be eating. Not everybody needs the same serving size, so it's important to consider your daily needs.

2. Measure your food. There are many different ways to understand serving sizes so we can have a better idea of what we are eating. If you're cooking at home (which is a great way to control portion size), you can make use of a kitchen scale, measuring cups, and meal prep containers to portion control your meals. When you're not at home, there are also several tips you can use, which I discuss later on in this post.

3. Meal prep. I love to meal prep because it is such a great way to help prepare you to succeed at your healthy goals. It helps to prep and cook balanced and healthy meals and full control over food portion sizes. The more you can plan ahead and make your well-balanced meal work for you, the better of you'll be.

4. Calculate your macros. It's important to get a good understanding of what your body needs in order to fully take advantage of portion control when trying to lose weight, gain weight, or maintain your weight. This one is a little tricky and does require some patience and learning. I'll cover how to calculate your macros later in this post so you can get started right away.

5. Fill up on veggies. Veggies and greens are always a good idea so make sure you enjoy them with every meal. They not only add valuable nutrients, but they also are filling and don't take up a bunch of calories, which allows you to better portion out your carbs and protein.

6. Go slow and steady. No one likes to be hungry all the time. It's a lifestyle that won't be satisfying and, thus, will likely fail when you are trying to lose weight. The best method for weight loss is gradual weight loss over time as part of a healthy, well-balanced lifestyle, not to restrict your calories so much that you're miserable. You can read more about my own personal struggle with weight and calories counting as well. That means you want to slowly reduce your portion sizes and your body gets used to the new levels. The more drastic you cut your food intake, the more your body and mind will fight you to give up.

7. Use smaller plates. There's something about finishing your plate that really makes a difference. I know it seems crazy, but using smaller plates will help you to feel like you're enjoying a full meal and will trick your brain into feeling satisfied. If you eat everything on your plate, but the plate is smaller, it will feel better than not eating everything on your plate with a larger plate. This is another reason I really like these glass meal prep containers — because I know I can eat everything in the container and it's still on track with my goals.

8. Drink more water. Did you know drinking water before a meal will help with portion control and will help you to lose weight faster? For realz! When we're dehydrated, we tend to eat more. So, drinking a glass of water before your meal actually helps because you'll be less tempted to eat a big portion size. If I know I've already eaten what my body needs and I start to feel hungry, I drink a glass of water and wait 30 minutes. If I'm still hungry, I know it's that I should eat a small snack, but often times, I'm no longer hungry – I was actually thirsty!

9. Eat slowly. It can be difficult at first to re-train yourself, but try to slow down your eating. The longer you take to eat your food, the more full you'll feel before you finish, which will help you eat what you need and not over-eat. Check out my tips for how to train yourself to eat more slowly later in this post.

10. Make a schedule. I found it really helpful to create a schedule with alarms on my phone that would let me know when breakfast, lunch, dinner, and snack times were. That way, I always had something to look forward to and knew I was just a little bit away, while I trained my body to not over-

eat anymore.

SERVING SIZE VERSUS PORTION SIZE: WHAT'S THE DIFFERENCE?

Learning how to measure food is very important and it will make portion control much easier. So, first, let's talk about the difference between serving size and portion size.

What Does Serving Size Mean?

Serving size is the recommended amount of a specific type of food. This is the recommended amount for a day, not for a meal. The serving size is what you will read on a nutrition label at the top for that product. Serving size, believe it or not, is actually NOT based on dietary needs to any large degree. The "serving size" we see at the top of nutrition labels (for example, 15 crackers, 8 oz., or 2 tbsp, etc.) was determined from the average amount Americans consumed in a single seating, based on federal food surveys between 1978 and 1988! Insane, right? The serving sizes listed on the Nutrition Facts label are NOT recommended serving sizes. By law, those serving sizes must actually be based on how much food people actually consume, and not on what they should eat. That means it is not very useful in understanding how much of that food we should be eating — you must understand that for yourself.

What Does Portion Size Mean?

The portion size is the actual amount of food you literally eat in one sitting. That means we need to understand serving sizes of our food and eat what our bodies require using portion control to lose weight and be healthy. It's also always important to remember your nutritional needs are likely very different than the ones of an average person, especially when you consider serving size wasn't even based on nutritional requirements.

Factors that can affect your daily caloric intake (and ideal portion size):

• level of physical activity (exercise increases your body's ability to burn calories)

• height

• age

• genetics

• diet (certain foods can increase or decrease your metabolism, which is what burns fat)

• gender

• drugs (certain drugs can help or hurt your metabolism)

• muscle mass (the more muscle you have, the more calories your body burns)

• body size

• hormonal imbalances

UNDERSTANDING MACROS

The first step in understanding how much food you should be eating to better succeed at portion control is to calculate your macros. What the heck are macros, you ask? Great question!

Read on and learn all about them and why they're so important for understanding portion control.

To start, all food is broken up into:

1. carbohydrates

2. protein, and

3. fat.

It's the combination of the three of these "macros" (short for "macronutrients") that make up what we call Calories.

- **Calories**

First and foremost, let's get one thing straight. A calorie, by itself, is not the evil thing you might thing it is. It is literally just a scientific way to measure energy. Calories aren't bad for you by themselves. Your body NEEDS calories for energy. But eating too many calories — and not burning enough of them off through activity — can lead to weight gain. In fact, it takes about 3,500 calories below your calorie needs to lose a pound of body fat. It takes approximately 3,500 calories above your calorie needs to gain a pound.

For the macros:

1. 1 g carbohydrate = 4 calories

2. 1 g protein = 4 calories

3. 1 g fat = 9 calories

This is why not all foods are created equal and why some contain more calories than others. It's also not just about how many calories you eat, it's about eating quality foods for your caloric intake.

Carbohydrates

Commonly referred to as "carbs," carbohydrates are in foods like bread, rice, and potatoes and they provide your body with heat and energy. There are three types of carbs:

4. Starches (found in vegetables, beans, grains, pasta, bread)

5. Sugars (found either naturally in fruits, milk, etc., or can be added to food, like with granulated sugar, brown sugar, honey, etc.)

6. Fibers (found in beans, fruit, veggies, whole grains, nuts, etc.)

Overall, the goal is to focus more on fiber and starches and limit sugars, especially those that aren't naturally occurring.

Protein

All of our organs, including skin, muscles, hair and nails are built from proteins. Additionally, hormones, the immune system, the digestive system, and our blood all rely on proteins to work correctly. Protein is, therefore, an essential part of our diet, vital to our development, and for proper functioning of the body. When we eat, our body breaks down the protein in our food in order to create the amino acids that it needs.

Foods high in protein:

- lean meat

- fish

- eggs

- dairy

- nuts

In order for protein to be broken down once we eat it, we NEED fat and carbohydrates to fuel the process. That's why having a well-balanced diet is so critical — you can't just eat protein and no fat or carbs — they all work together.

• **Fat**

Fat makes food taste better and makes us feel full longer, but what does it do for our bodies? Believe it or not, fat is also an essential part of our diet and nutrition, meaning we literally cannot live without it. While our bodies require small amounts of "good fat" to function and help prevent disease, a lot of diets contain far more fat than the body needs. Too much fat, especially too much of the wrong type of fat, can cause serious health problems, including obesity, high blood pressure, and high cholesterol, all of which can lead to a greater risk of heart disease.

Types of fat:

• **Unsaturated Fat** – Unsaturated fats are generally considered the best kind of fat. Unsaturated fats come from vegetable sources and are encouraged as part of a healthy diet. These fats help reduce heart disease, lower cholesterol levels and have other health benefits.

- **Saturated Fat** – Generally, saturated fats come from animal sources (meat, dairy, eggs etc.), and are usually solid at room temperature. Common sources of saturated fat include: Beef, Lamb, Pork, Dairy products made from whole milk (milk, cheese, butter), poultry skin, palm oil, etc.

- **Hydrogenated / Trans Fat** – Almost exclusively manufactured and are used in many processed foods. They are linked to an increased risk of high cholesterol levels and coronary heart disease. These are the worst of all fats when it comes to health. Manufacturers use trans fats because it increases the shelf life of fat and makes the fat harder at room temperature.

Understanding what macros are and why we need them is very helpful for approaching portion control — it's the "why" behind a well-balanced meal, and what that means for our bodies.

HOW TO CALCULATE MACROS

So...how do you calculate your macros? While you can calculate it yourself using a formula, I recommend using the IIFYM calculator (IIFYM stands for "If It Fits Your Macros"), which helps you take activity level, goals, and many other factors into account. It is very quick to calculate and will provide you with how many calories you should eat each day, based on your goals, as well as how many grams of protein, fat, and carbohydrates to eat each day to reach your goals, whether that's to lose, gain, or maintain weight.

Once you have a base-line understanding of what macros your body requires, you can break down the foods you're eating and control the portions to best fit your macros. It can seem a little overwhelming to start, but it becomes more second nature the more you learn what makes up your food.

HOW TO EAT SLOWLY FOR BETTER PORTION CONTROL

One of the reasons we tend to eat too much is because we don't pay attention to what and how much we're eating and how fast we're doing it. Multitasking is not good for portion control, peeps. So try mindful eating. This means: slow down and experience your meal. For instance, did you know it can take your body up to 20 minutes to feel full? So, if you devour your meal within 4 minutes, there's no way your body will feel full, and you'll eat more than you need. If we eat too fast, we will over-eat and not feel satisfied from a meal that should actually be totally satisfying.

To learn how to eat slowly, try the following...

• chew each bite 15-20 times;

• don't shovel food in your mouth, take small bite after small bite;

• eat at the table and focus on your meal, not on other things (don't watch TV or stay in front of your PC, you might end up eating more if you don't pay attention to your food);

• be aware of how full you are and stop if you feel satisfied (learn the difference in how you feel when "satisfied" versus "full");

• save extra food for later if necessary (you don't need to eat everything).

Yes, life is busy and hectic, but the more we can practice mindful eating, the better off we will be – food will taste better, we will feel nourished, and we'll lose weight along the way!

SHOULD I KEEP A FOOD JOURNAL?

Another great idea for those just getting started learning how to portion control is to keep a food journal. A food journal is a great way to manage food portion sizes and to make sure they follow the portion sizes we've determined, based on our individual needs.

So, how do you keep a food journal or diary? You can choose to either keep track using an app or on a notepad. The idea is to track everything you eat, including portion sizes, each day. This will help provide you with a baseline for how much you're currently eating and to keep track of your goals each day. I prefer the MyFitnessPal app, but there are many, many free and paid options out there.

A word of caution: While I do believe tracking your meals is a fantastic way to create a baseline or starting point, and to reel in what you're eating to better understand why you may or may not be losing weight, I recommend limiting the amount of time you keep a diary. Over time, you'll be able to understand portions on your own, which is ideal to avoid becoming obsessed with every single calorie in your diary — trust me, I've been there. Once you've tracked your food for about a month, you should have a pretty good understanding of what portions you should be eating. The better you can trust yourself with your food choices, the more healthy of a lifestyle it will be. This is also what makes eating clean a fantastic choice because you don't have so many empty calories of sugar and processed fats.

HOW TO CUT DOWN PORTIONS WITHOUT FEELING HUNGRY

If you're worried that eating smaller portions will make you feel hungry all the time, I totally understand. I think everyone's been on "that diet" where you felt like you were starving from meal to meal, only to finally eat another meal that wasn't filling enough. This can cause un-needed stress, and is exactly what we want to avoid. So, take it one step at a time. Use this post to find out the ideal macros for you, then start to focus on your food portion sizes. Take note of the portions you're currently eating — are they way too big? Try reducing them slightly, but do it progressively. If you want to be successful at the portion control, treat it like a marathon, not a sprint, and set yourself up for success.

Here are some more portion control tips to help you feel satisfied (not starving!):

• Overload on veggies and greens and follow more strict portions for higher calorie/fat foods, like carbs, proteins, and fats;

• Fill up on water as much as possible – remember your body tricks you that you're hungry when you may actually be thirsty;

• Put aside a part of your meal for later. If, in 20 minutes you're still hungry, finish eating. If not, save for later in the fridge.

• Eat snacks! Snacking between meals will make eating smaller portions much easier. Just make sure those snacks are healthy and good for you.

• Make sure you're eating the right macros. make use of healthy fats, proteins, and complex carbs so you're not running on fumes.

• Ask yourself if you're really hungry or if you just THINK you're hungry because you're used to eating more. This will be a gradual process you'll need to learn.

HOW TO EAT SMALLER PORTIONS AT RESTAURANTS

Portion control at restaurants is very tricky, especially nowadays when restaurants serve extra-large portions. It is definitely manageable, though, so don't worry. I still like to eat out from time to time, but I'm able to keep my portion sizes under control. Here's how you can do it, too:

• Check the meal portion size or ask the staff – order something that is close to your ideal food portion sizes;

- Ask for a half order (they can even box it for you ahead of time so you never see it!);

- Use the 50/25/25 rule for each meal (50% carbs / 25% fat / 25% protein) to feel full and have more energy;

- Take leftovers to go if you really crave something that comes in an extra-large portion;

- Split the meal with someone – you can split the appetizers, the main dish, and even the dessert;

• Eat until you are satisfied and take the rest to go – don't overeat just to finish the portion!

• Remember to go heavy on the greens and always ask for veggies as a side.

• Drink your water so you feel full.

These tips will help you to eat smaller portions at restaurants for sure.

PORTION CONTROL AS A LIFESTYLE, NOT JUST A DIET

I think it's best to remember that portion control is an active choice you make as an investment in your healthy lifestyle and overall wellness journey.

Portion control can help you lose weight and also keep weight off, and it's all part of the process of controlling what foods you're eating with clean eating. Hopefully, you'll find how good it feels to be in control of your food (instead of at war) and aware of what, how much, and when you're eating. Mindful eating and informed choices – this is the power of portion control. And I'm sure you'll notice the long-term, positive effects along the way!

• MEAL PREP IDEAS FOR PORTION CONTROL

Now that you're on board with portion control, I'm betting you could use some helpful recipes to get you started. Here are some of my absolute favorite meal prep recipes because they are well-balanced, delicious, filling, easy, and, of course, allow you to portion control your food!